The Guru Method

Biology

For information contact:

GSMS Education Pty Ltd
P.O Box 3848
Marsfield NSW
2122
Australia

How to use The Guru Method Biology Manual

The Biology Questions in Section III of the GAMSAT are based on the same problem solving principles as the Chemistry and the Physics sections. Questions require candidates to dissect passages and diagrams rather than to rote learn and regurgitate facts.

The breadth of topics that theoretically could be examined is endless. It is for this reason that a lot of theoretical material is purposefully skipped in this manual. The manual consists of material that only gives a BRIEF overview of important ideas and topics. It is imperative that you overcome what is called "information overload" in biology and learn to focus on the techniques and methodology of answering GAMSAT questions.

In general, biology questions will be either one of two sorts.

1. "Lone standing" questions will test you on your factual knowledge
2. More commonly, a series of questions will be asked in relation to a passage and a diagram.

Reading graphs and interpreting diagrams is of the utmost importance and definitely more important than rote learning "factual" material from a typical university textbook. Unlike chemistry and Physics there are very few "QUICK FACTS" contained in this manual as I feel that they are of little benefit.

Probably the most important concepts to grasp in BIOLOGY are graph reading and interpretation. If you can significantly improve your skills in this area, it will be of a great advantage in answering biology questions in the GAMSAT.

I wish you the best of luck and hope that this manual serves you well.

Table of Contents

Chapter 1: **Demystifying graphs and charts**

In the GAMSAT, there will be a lot of questions requiring the interpretation of graphs, charts and tables. One of the most important skills is to be able to interpret graphs quickly.

Tip: **Know how to read graphs well. Most Biology questions will involve reading a graph or interpreting a diagram.**

Graphs are of four basic types:
1. Pie charts
2. Bar graphs
3. Line graphs
4. XY-plots

The type chosen depends on the characteristics of the data displayed.

Pie chart

Pie charts explain the relationship of a part to the whole. Pie charts are not used as frequently as other types.

Table 1 below shows data from a group of hospital patients who have recently been diagnosed as hypertensive.

Observations

Table I: Showing age distribution

Age (yrs)	Males	Females
30-39	4	1
40-49	8	1
50-59	15	7
60-65	3	1
Total	30 (75%)	10 (25%)

Table 1

The pie chart in Fig 1 explains the sex distribution. Note that the area of the circle takes the same proportion of the data. That is 25% female means, one-fourth of the diagram (marked in black). Similarly, 75% of the males contribute 75% of the circle.

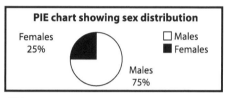

Fig. 1.

The pie chart in Fig 2 provides the ratio of the severity or the grade of the hypertension. 30% of them are moderate and 70% of them are mild.

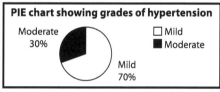

Fig. 2.

Bar graph

Bar graphs are display data using a horizontal or vertical rectangular bar that levels off at the appropriate level.

The characteristics of bar graphs are:

- They make comparisons between different variables very easy to see.
- They clearly show trends in data, meaning that they show how one variable is affected as the other rises or falls.
- Given one variable, the value of the other can be easily determined.

he figure given below depicts fat content in different types of cheese. One who wishes to reduce
1eir fat intake can go for cottage dry cheese.

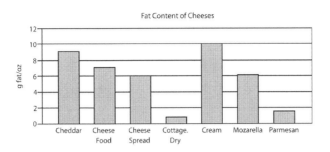

ie charts are effective for displaying the relative frequencies of a small number of categories. Bar
raphs are better when there are more than just a few categories and for comparing two or more
istributions. See the example below between a pie chart and a bar graph.

dvanced bar graphs

3ar graphs can also compare relationships between related data sets.

Illustrative questions

Question (1-3).

The bar graph given below depicts the percentage of different diseases in a population.
Simultaneously it shows the distribution within male and female.

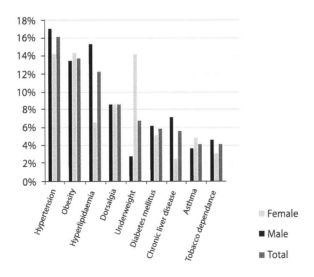

1. The disease which has the same distribution between the male and female is

    A. Obesity,
    B. Dorsalgia,
    C. Underweight,
    D. Asthma

2. The disease which has the largest variation between the male and female is

    A. Obesity,
    B. Dorsalgia,
    C. Underweight,
    D. Asthma

3. Which of the three diseases together contribute more than 40 % of the female population?

    A. Obesity, dorsalgia and underweight
    B. Hypertension, obesity and underweight
    C. Obesity, dorsalgia and asthma
    D. Dorsalgia, underweight and asthma

Solution

Question 1.
Step 1: Intepreting the question
Key words are same distribution, male and female.

Step 2: Gathering data
To read the graph, look at the height of each bar and read off the y-axis.

Step 3: Solution
The bars that have equal height for male and female is B.

Question 2.

Step 1: Intepreting the question
Key words are largest variation, male and female.

Steps 2 and 3: Gathering data and solution
Look for the graph that has the largest difference in the height of the columns between male and female. The answer is C.

Question 3.

Step 1: Intepreting the question
Key words are three diseases, 40%, female.

Steps 2 and 3: Gathering data and solution
Read off the graph the percentages for each disease listed and add together. Answer B has roughly 14% +14% +14% which is more than 40%. Therefore the answer is B.

Line graphs

Line graphs compare two variables. Each variable is plotted along an axis. A line graph has a vertical axis and a horizontal axis.

Some of the characteristics of line graphs are that:

- They are good at showing specific values of data, meaning that given one variable the other can easily be determined.
- They show trends in data clearly, meaning that they visibly show how one variable is affected by the other as it increases or decreases.
- They enable the viewer to make predictions about the results of data not yet recorded.

Illustrative questions

Question 1.

The graphs shown below depict the data collected from a longitudinal study of the growth of a large number of children. Separate graphs are provided for boys and girls.

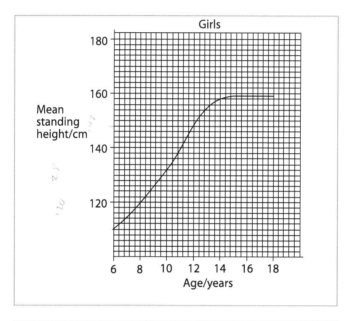

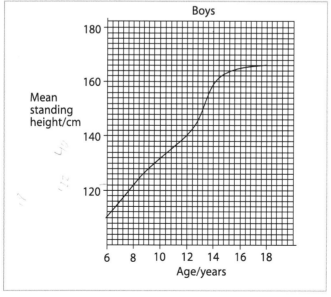

1. The difference in growth rate between boys and girls from age 8 to 12 is

rate = $\frac{y}{x}$ ic he gradient

A. 3.0cm/year
B. 4.0cm/year
C. 2.0cm/year
D. 5.0cm/year

Tip: In GAMSAT you may have to read the graph in many questions. Your success depends on how quickly you can grasp the concepts you are reading and converting this into the required data. Once you know the basics, this is not a big issue. You should not be perplexed by seeing some variables which you are seeing for the first time in your life.

Question 2.

The figure shows the nitrogen content in a plant as it grew to maturity.

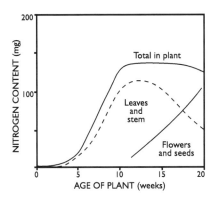

2. When was the fastest uptake of nitrogen for the whole plant?

A. 0-5 weeks
B. 5-10 weeks
C. 10-15 weeks
D. 15-20 weeks

Solution

Question 1.

Step 1: Intepreting the question

Key words are: rate, boys and girls and 8 to 12 years age. When you encounter the word: "rate", think rise/run or units of specified measurement per unit of time. With the word "difference", think of minus (-). So the question basically asks what is the rate of growth of girls between the ages of 8 to 12 minus the rate for boys in the same time period.

Steps 2 and 3: Gathering data and solution

Read the Graph. Where does the y axis intercept at years 8 and 12 for both boys and girls.
Boys: (8, 122), (12, 140) therefore rise over run $\Rightarrow$ 18/4 cm/year = 4.5cm/year
Girls: (8,120), (12, 150) therefore rise over run $\Rightarrow$ 30/4cm/year = 7.5cm/year
Difference= 7.5-4.5=3.0cm/year

Therefore: A

Question 2.

Step 1: Intepreting the question
Key word is 'rate'. What is the rate?

Steps 2 and 3: Gathering data and solution
Graph- Rise over Run = rate
Steepest area of the graph s between 5 to 10 weeks. Therefore: B

XY-Plots

XY-Plots are similar to line graphs in that they use horizontal and vertical axes to plot data points However, they have a very specific purpose. XY-plots show how much one variable is affected by another. The relationship between two variables is called their correlation.

XY-Plots usually consist of a large body of data. The closer the data points come when plotted to making a straight line, the higher the correlation between the two variables, or the stronger the relationship.

Illustrative questions

Question (1-2).

The diagram below shows the daily energy expenditure of a number of animals.

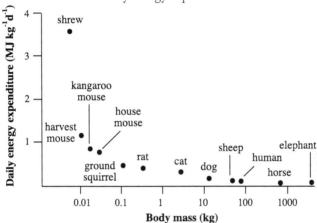

1. Which animal would have the highest energy requirements per day?

    A. Mouse
    B. Sheep
    C. Horse
    D. Dog

2. From the graph, which statement is correct?

    A. The higher the body mass of an animal the higher the quality of food it requires
    B. The higher the body mass of the animal the more energy it requires per body mass unit.
    C. The lower the body mass of an animal the more energy it requires per body mass unit.
    D. Daily energy requirement is a function of body mass

Question (3-4).

The presences of Stomatal pores in plants are an adaptation to special conditions of life on the land. When pores are open, CO_2 can readily diffuse through to photosynthetic cells and O_2 can diffuse out. The diameters of the stomatal pores are very small and it is very difficult to gauge their efficiency directly. It is simpler and easier to study the changes in the stomatal pores indirectly by measuring the total water loss from the leaves which can indicate whether the pores are open or shut. The figure below shows the apertures of a Native Australian Tree growing in dry conditions. Measurements were made of the degree of opening of the pores over a 24-hour period. The weather had been dry and little water existed in the soil. The stomata were only opened for a brief period. The opening and closing of these pores regulates the diffusion of gases into or out of the leaf. CO_2 is needed for photosynthesis therefore the stomatal pores must open. Closure of the stomatal pores restricts this water loss when water is in short supply. The graph below shows the typical stomatal aperture opening of an Australian plant in a very dry climate.

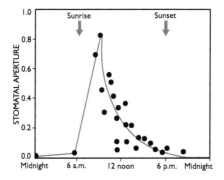

3. In terms of the opening mechanism of stomatal pores, what does the graph suggest?

   A. That Sunlight has a major effect on the diameter of the pores also having an immediate effect.
   B. Time of day is the major factor that determines the stomatal opening aperture
   C. Aperture is a function of on the weather conditions
   D. CO_2 content in the air has a major effect on the opening of the aperture

4. How would you expect this behaviour of stomatal opening to compare with that of a plant in well-watered soil?

   A. Stomata diameter becomes wider
   B. Stomata opens longer between sunset and sunrise
   C. It stays the same
   D. Need more information.

Solution

Question 1.

Step 1: Intepreting the question
Key words are "highest energy requirements". This means total energy requirement of the animal. This is not to be confused with the highest rate of energy requirement per unit mass of the animal.

Step 2: Gathering data
The four choices given are mouse, sheep, horse and dog. In answering this question, we need to keep in mind the size of the animal and the energy expenditure per kg. Therefore, the larger the animal, the more energy requirement, and the smaller the animal, the higher the energy requirement per kg of body mass. Also note that the x-axis (body mass) is in logarithmic scale, while the y-axis (energy expenditure) is linear.

Step 3: Solution
The horse has nearly 100 and 50 times greater mass than the dog and sheep respectively, but maybe only 2 times lower energy expenditure per kg. Therefore, the horse uses 50 to 25 times more energy than the dog and sheep respectively. The horse is nearly 10000 times heavier than the mouse, but has around 10 times lower energy expenditure. Therefore answer is horse (c).

> **Tip:**   Always skim the answers before trying to gauge an answer. It may save you a lot of time.

Question 2.

Step 1: Intepreting the question
Key words are "correct" and "statement".

Steps 2 and 3: Gathering data and solution
The graph only provides information about daily energy expenditure versus body mass. Therefore **A** cannot be concluded from this data. With increasing body mass, daily energy expenditure drops, there B is incorrect.

Hence C is the correct answer.

Question 3.

Step 1: Intepreting the question
Key Words: Opening mechanism, diameter of pore, graph, suggest. When words such as "suggest" occur, it implies that the answer is not definite but asks the reader to pick the most suitable option. In this case the question asks us to form a link between the peaks and trough of the graph and the other variables in the graph.

Step 2 - Gathering Data
In the graph we can see a line that shifts throughout the day. Always look at the variables and assessing what they really mean. Here we are looking at the "stomatal aperture", "time of day" and also "sunrise" and "sunset". Sift through the passage and find the relevant data.

Step 3 - Solution
This is where the reasoning comes in. Look at the four answers. The last two options C and D are automatically out because the question asks the relevance to the graph. So it comes down to A and B. Out of these two, we must pick which one is the most accurate even though both sound true. B says that time of day is the factor but although there is a peak after sunrise, there is no definite pattern that the graph suggest. A is the more accurate. Therefore A

> **Tip:** Always check the relevance of answers to the question. Often an answer may be factually correct but is unrelated to the question.

Question 4.

Step 1: Intepreting the question
Key Words: expect, compare, stomatal opening. The question asks to extrapolate data given in the introduction of the question and apply it to the graph.

Steps 2 and 3: Gathering data and solution
In the introduction it states that water is in short supply, and that the plant conserves water by closing its stomata. However, the stomata have to open during the day for photosynthesis. Hence during periods of greater water supply, it is reasonable to suggest that the stomata stay open longer during night time, as no water has to be conserved (B), however, we have no data to confirm this fact. Similar reasoning for C. Hence we need more information, and the correct answer is D.

Chapter 2: Eukaryotic and Prokaryotic Organisms

> **Tip:** This material is a general summary of cell types. There are very rarely any direct questions on this. Questions will normally be of an indirect nature. Consistent with the other parts of the manual is the brevity of topic dissection. For a more comprehensive overview, please consult a biology textbook.

Key concepts: Prokaryotic Cells

- Have the simplest overall structure.
- Bounded by a lipid bi-layer membrane, but does not contain any internal membrane-bound organelles.
- Contains a region rich in DNA called a nucleoid and contains a circular molecule of DNA which is the cells genetic material, or genome.
- Surrounding the nucleoid is a region of cytoplasm rich in ribosomes, small protein-RNA structures which do the job of synthesizing proteins
- Surrounding the plasma membrane is a cell wall
- Flagella (surface appendages) are used for locomotion. One of the more surprising aspects of cell structure is the way that DNA molecules are packaged into cells.
- In the nucleoid, the DNA is both compacted so as to fit within the bacterium, and yet is still accessible to the machinery necessary both to read the genetic instructions (synthesize RNA) and to copy the DNA (replicate).

Key concepts: Eukaryotic cells

- Much more complex than prokaryotic cells
- Much of the cell is taken up by subcellular organelles bound by their own membranes (analogous to the plasma membrane surrounding the cell)
- Have a nucleus which contains all of the cell's DNA
- "Eukaryote" means "true nucleus" while "prokaryote" means "before the nucleus".
- The problem of packaging DNA is greater in eukaryotes.

Key concepts: Membrane Traffic

Transport of molecules across a membrane may be active or passive
- For net movement of molecules across a membrane, two features are required:
    - (1) The molecule must be able to cross a hydrophobic barrier
    - (2) An energy source must power the movement.
- Lipophilic molecules can pass through a membrane's hydrophobic interior by simple diffusion. These molecules will *move down* their concentration gradients.
- Polar or charged molecules require proteins to *form passages* through the hydrophobic barrier.

Key concepts: Passive transport or facilitated diffusion vs. active transport

- Passive transport occurs when an ion or polar molecule moves down its concentration gradient.
- If a molecule moves against a concentration gradient, an external energy source is required; this movement is referred to as *active transport* and results in the generation of concentration gradients. Concentration gradients are a commonly used form of energy in all organisms.

Key concepts: Osmosis

- Osmosis is a special term used for the diffusion of water through cell membranes.
- Although water is a polar molecule, it is *able to pass through the lipid bi-layer* of the plasma membrane.
- *Water passes by diffusion from a region of higher to a region of lower concentration. Note that this refers to the concentration of water, NOT the concentration of any solutes present in the water.*
- Water is never transported actively; that is, it never moves against its concentration gradient. However, the concentration of water can be altered by the active transport of solutes and in this way the movement of water in and out of the cell can be controlled.

Example: the reabsorption of water from the kidney tubules back into the blood depends on the water following behind the active transport of Na^+.

GAMSAT Style Questions

Tip: **Understand the Key concepts for Osmosis, questions will frequently arise in the GAMSAT that will require you to have an understanding of this topic.**

Question 1.

Normally, in the process of osmosis, the net flow of water molecules into or out of the cell depends upon differences in the

A. concentration of water molecules inside and outside the cell

B. concentration of enzymes on either side of the cell membrane

C. rate of molecular motion on either side of the cell membrane

D. rate of movement of insoluble molecules inside the cell

Question 2.

It is normally necessary to give patients large volumes of fluids after extreme dehydration or blood loss. One example of fluid commonly used is normal saline, which is a 0.9% NaCl solution, and has an osmolarity similar to extracellular fluid. On the basis that red blood cells are water permeable, but impermeable to Na^+ and Cl^- ions, a red blood cell that is immersed in a saline solution which has 2.0% NaCl will

A. shrink, as the osmotic pressure forces the water out of the cell

B. swell, as the osmotic pressure forces water into the cell

C. stay the same, as osmotic pressure has no effect over the red blood cell's membrane

D. die, as 2% NaCl is toxic and will cause cell membrane disruption.

Question (3-5).

Diffusion is the net movement of molecules of a substance from a region of their higher concentration to a region of their lower concentration. The average distance a molecule, travels in time 't' is proportional to the "square root of time". Net movement means there are more molecules moving in one direction than in the opposite direction. Opening a bottle of perfume in a room will result in the gradual diffusion of the perfume from the region of higher concentration (the bottle) out into the room. Diffusion will continue until the perfume has a more or less uniform concentration throughout the bottle and room.

A differentially permeable membrane is one that some molecules can pass through, while other molecules cannot. Osmosis is the diffusion of a solvent through a differentially permeable membrane.

3. A semi permeable membrane separates a solution that is 0.012M glucose from one that is 0.250 M glucose. On which of this solution must pressure be applied to prevent a net flow of water through the membrane?

     A. On the 0.012 M solution

     B. On the 0.250 M solution

     C. Equal pressure on both the solutions

     D. The pressure on 0.012 M solution should be doubled of the pressure on 0.250M solution

4. If 0.1 molar solution of glucose (MW=180) is separated from 0.1 molar solution of cane sugar (MW=342) by a semi permeable membrane, then which one of the following statements is CORRECT?

     A. Water will flow from glucose solution into cane sugar solution

     B. Cane sugar will flow across the membrane into glucose solution

     C. Glucose will flow across the membrane into cane sugar solution

     D. There will be no net movement across the semi permeable membrane

5. A drop of colored water is dropped into a glass of clear water. It was observed that the radius of the colored water blob grows from 1 mm to 2mm in 5 s . Assume that the rate of diffusion is independent of concentration Approximately how much longer will it take to grow to 4 mm?

     A. 2 minutes

     B. 20 seconds

     C. 1 minute

     D. 40 seconds.

Solution

Question 1.

Step 1: Intepreting the question
Key Words: osmosis and net flow.

Steps 2 and 3: Gathering data and solution
Osmosis is the diffusion of water across a membrane and is a passive process. Therefore, movement occurs due to a concentration gradient set up on either side of the membrane. If there is more water inside the cell than outside, water tends to move out. Therefore answer is A.

Question 2.

Step 1: Intepreting the question
Key Word: Osmolarity. The question asks what effect a hypertonic solution has on a red blood cell.

Steps 2 and 3: Gathering data and solution
The introductory statement indicates that a red blood cell is impermeable to both Na^+ and Cl^- ions. 2% saline has an osmolarity higher than found *in vivo* which has been stated to be 0.9%. Therefore the solution is *hypertonic*. Because the concentrations of ions are higher in the extracellular solution, water will pass through the membrane from the cytosol. A net loss of water from the cell causes the cell to *shrink*. Therefore answer is A.

Question 3

Step 1: Intepreting the question
The question implies that if water is placed in one of the solution then it will flow to the other side because of the osmotic pressure. It is asking from which side does the water go to so you can prevent it from entering in.

Step 2: Gathering data
Osmosis involves the flow of molecules from a low concentration side to the higher concentration side. There are two sides of the solution with different concentrations of glucose. 0.25M is obviously more concentrated then the 0.12M. So if water is added, there will be a higher concentration of water in the 0.12 M solution and will flow towards the 0.25M solution.

Step 3: Solution
As a result to prevent a net flow of water through the membrane, pressure must be applied on the concentrated solution side i.e. 0.250 M. The answer is B

Question 4

Step 1: Intepreting the question
Always scan the answers. Looking at the answers, the question is asking "which substance flows where?"

Step 2: Gathering data
In terms of osmosis the relevant data we need to know the concentration of the solutions. Here the concentrations are both given in the question. This is trick question as it gives the molecular weight of the compounds which are of no real use for finding the concentration.

Step 3: Solution
As both the solutions have the same molarities, there will be no osmosis, no net flow across the semi permeable membrane. The answer is D

Question 5

Step 1: Intepreting the question
The question is asking for the difference in time t from the time it takes to grow from 2mm to 5mm

Step 2: Gathering data
The passage tells us that the distance is proportional to the square root of the time taken to travel the distance.

Step 3: Solution
Diffusion: Average distance a molecule travels in time t, $x = \sqrt{2Dt}$

$$x_1 = \sqrt{2Dt_1}, x_2 = \sqrt{2Dt_2} \Rightarrow \frac{x_2}{x_1} = \sqrt{\frac{t_2}{t_1}} \Rightarrow t_2 = t_1 \left(\frac{x_2}{x_1}\right)^2$$

$$t_2 = 5\left(\frac{4-2}{2-1}\right)^2 s = 20s$$

Note: $\sqrt{2D}$ is a factor of proportionality and cancels itself out by the last line.

Chapter 3: **Cell Division**

> *Tip:* **Questions will very rarely be asked in this topic in the GAMSAT, please have a basic understanding of the concepts here.**

Key concepts: Cell Cycle and Mitosis

1. Stages of the cell cycle – Figure 1

- The cell cycle is a set of events that culminates in cell growth and division into two daughter cells.
- Non-dividing cells are not considered to be in the cell cycle.
- The stages pictured in Figure 1, are G1-S-G2-M.
    - o G1 stage stands for "Gap 1".
    - o S stage stands for "Synthesis". This is the stage when DNA replication occurs.
    - o G2 stage stands for "Gap 2".
    - o M stage stands for "mitosis", and is when nuclear (chromosomes separate) and cytoplasmic (cytokinesis) division occur. Mitosis is further divided into 4 phases.

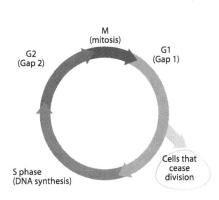

Figure 1

Chapter 4: Enzymatic Activity & Metabolic pathways

Key concepts: Metabolic pathways

A *metabolic pathway* is a series of chemical reactions within a cell, catalysed by enzymes, which either results in the formation of a product to be used or stored by the cell (metabolic sink), or the initiation of another metabolic pathway.

Most metabolic pathways have common properties:

- They are irreversible, usually because the first step is a committed step that only runs in one direction.
- The pathways are regulated, usually by feedback inhibition.
- *Anabolic* and *catabolic* pathways in eukaryotes are separated by either compartmentation or by the use of different enzymes and co-factors.

> Tip: It is not critical to memorise all these concepts. We will discuss only Glycolysis at this stage to introduce you to the basics. You will never be asked on any of this knowledge directly, i.e. how many ATPs does the glycolysis produce in one cycle? It is more important to understand the logic and process behind the basic mechanism. Understand how an enzyme works. Understand what a metabolic pathway's purpose is. Use what is given in the questions, such as the glycolysis cycle to understand the concept of metabolic pathways.

> Tip: If you have no previous university level biochemistry experience, look up Glycolysis in a textbook just to gain a general understanding of the concept. There is no need to delve deeper into this topic. Once you understand the basics, you will be able to apply the information given to answer the questions in the GAMSAT!

Key concepts: Major metabolic pathways

Several distinct but linked metabolic pathways are used by cells to transfer the energy released by breakdown of fuel molecules to ATP:

1. Glycolysis
2. Anaerobic respiration
3. Krebs' cycle
4. Oxidative phosphorylation

→Quick Facts: Glycolysis

- Glycolysis is the initial metabolic pathway of carbohydrate catabolism.
- Glycolysis is the most universal process by which cells of all types derive energy from sugars. It is not the most efficient, but glycolysis proper is completely anaerobic; that is, oxygen is not required.

Output of Glycolysis
- Glycolysis converts one molecule of glucose into two molecules of pyruvate, along with "reducing equivalents" in the form of the co-enzyme NADH.

The global reaction of glycolysis is:

$$\text{Glucose} + 2\text{ NAD}^+ + 2\text{ ADP} + 2\text{ P}_i \rightarrow 2\text{ NADH} + 2\text{ pyruvate} + 2\text{ ATP} + 2\text{ H}_2\text{O} + 4\text{ H}^+$$

- For simple fermentations, the metabolism of 1 molecule of glucose has a net yield of 2 molecules of ATP.
- Cells performing respiration synthesize much more ATP but this is not considered part of glycolysis.

Location
- In eukaryotes glycolysis takes place within the cytosol of the cell (as opposed to the mitochondria, where reactions more closely connected to aerobic metabolism occur).
- Glucose gets into the cell through facilitated diffusion. In some tissues such as skeletal muscle, insulin stimulates this process.

> **Tip:** You do not need to have a detailed understanding of the above concepts. Focus on understanding the fundamentals.

Key concepts: Enzyme kinetics

Definition of Enzyme: Any of several complex proteins that are produced by cells and acted as catalysts in specific biochemical reactions.

Inhibition
- Substances that reduce an enzyme's activity in this way are known as inhibitors.
- Most inhibitors are substances that structurally resemble their enzyme's substrate but either does not react or react very slowly compared to substrate.

Competitive inhibitor

- A substance that competes directly with a normal substrate for an enzymatic-binding site is known as a competitive inhibitor.
- Such an inhibitor usually resembles the substrate to the extent that it specifically binds to the active site but differs from it so as to be non-reactive.

A competitive inhibitor therefore acts by reducing the concentration of free enzyme available for substrate binding.

GAMSAT Style Questions

> **Tip:** Do not get bogged down by the jargon in the questions. Often, these questions turn out to be simple mathematics problems. This is true for many questions in the GAMSAT. Once you recognize the patterns you will be able to maximize your performance.

Question 1.

The concentration of a substrate, enzyme and competitive inhibitor during the course of a reaction greatly affect the reaction rate. The initial velocity V_o, of the reaction can be expressed as

$$V_o = \frac{V_{max}[S]}{\alpha K_m + [S]}$$

Where:
α is a function of the inhibitor concentration,
K_m is Michaelis Constant,
V_{max} is the maximum velocity of the reaction and
S is the substrate concentration.

K_m is defined as the substrate concentration which produces ½ the maximum reaction velocity.

The graph below is the hyperbolic plot of the above equation for various values of α.

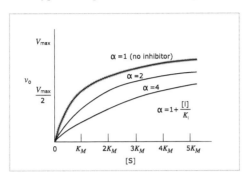

1. What would the value of α be if the substrate concentration [S] approached ∞ and V_0 approached V_{max}?

    A. $\alpha = 1$

    B. $\alpha = 2$

    C. $\alpha = 4$

    D. For all values of α

Question 2.

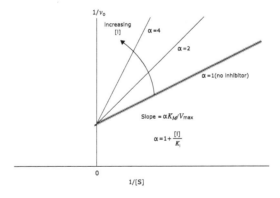

Above is a graph representing plots for the values of 1/Vo and 1/[S] for a particular enzymatic reaction with a competitive inhibitor and of which α is a function. Using the above equation for reaction velocity, what values of α is the 1/[S] intercept of the above plot greatest (consider K_m and V_0 having positive values)?

    A. $\alpha = 1$

    B. $\alpha = 2$

    C. $\alpha = 4$

    D. For all values of α

Solution

Question 1.

Step 1: Intepreting the question
Key words: substrate and infinity. The question asks what effect does an inhibitor have on maximal velocity of a reaction.

Steps 2 and 3: Gathering data and solution
An antagonist competes with the substrate to bind to the enzyme. Hence, the greater the concentration of the inhibitor, the slower the velocity of the reaction. However, when the concentration of the substrate approach infinity, then the speed of the reaction approaches V_{max}. Hence, the presence of the inhibitor is inconsequential, and it would be equivalent to having no inhibitor present ($\alpha=1$). Hence, answer is A.

Question 2.

Step 1: Intepreting the question
The question asks at what concentrations of effect does an inhibitor have on maximal velocity of a reaction.

Step 2 and 3 - Gathering Data and Solution
The higher the level of inhibitor present, the greater the concentration of substrate needed to have an equivalent reaction rate. The highest $1/[S]$ intercept would occur at the lowest concentration of substrate. From the graph, when the lines are extrapolated to hit the x-axis ($1/[S]$), it can be seen that higher values of α result in higher values of $[S]$, and hence smaller values of $1/[S]$. Therefore, the highest value of $1/[S]$ is when $[S]$ is smallest. Smaller values of substrate are needed when no inhibitor is present, hence the highest value of $1/[S]$ is when $\alpha =1$. The answer is A.

Chapter 5: **Muscular and skeletal systems**

Key concepts: Muscular and Skeletal systems

- The human body is supported by 206 bones that connect together to make the skeleton
- The skeleton is held together by joints by ligaments
- Movements of skeleton are effected by muscles which are attached to the bones by tendons
- Muscle is a flexible fibrous material which surrounds the skeleton
- Movements are produced by tensing the muscle which cause it to become shorter, fatter and pull on the bone, to restore the muscle to it's original position there is always an opposing muscle acting in antagonism

> **Tip:** Often in GAMSAT questions, Physics questions will masquerade as Biology questions. Often you will be asked to find mathematical expressions of bodily functions through the use of Physics formulae. We have included some of these questions in the Physics manual as well below in the GAMSAT Style Questions. The purpose of these is to develop your perceptive skills, cut through the verbosity and find the answer in the simplest manner possible.

GAMSAT Style Questions

Question (1 – 2).

In the diagram below the force generated by the bicep muscle is 1,050 N. The distance from the point of applied force to the axis of rotation of the elbow joint is shown as 4.0×10^{-2} m. A device for measuring force reads 127 N at a distance of 3.3×10^{-2} m from the axis of rotation at the elbow.

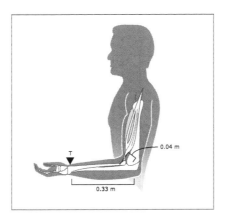

1. The torque developed about the elbow joint is

    A. 42 N -m
    B. 26150 N- m
    C. 794545 N- m
    D. 0 N- m

2. When the upper limb is assessed in a mechanical device, the torque developed is

    A. 26150 N- m
    B. 794545 N- m
    C. 0 N- m
    D. same as in the above case.

Question (3 – 4).

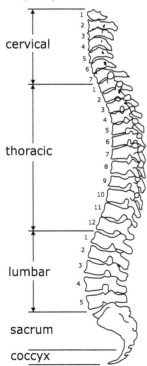

A study conducted on compressive strength of **VERTEBRAE AND INTERVERTEBRAL DISCS** of two bodies (Body A, B) have yielded the results as shown in the table below.

The different parts of the **VERTEBRAE AND INTERVERTEBRAL DISCS** are provided in the figure to the left. The first letter of the vertebrae part is used for identifying the body part in the tables shown below (e.g. C5 for fifth division of cervical).

Body A

Vertebrae	Compressive strength	
	Min. Value	Max. value
T-8	540	640
T-9	610	720
T-10	660	800
T-11	720	860
T-12	690	900
L-1	720	900
L-2	800	990
L-3	900	1100
L-4	900	1200
L-5	1000	1300

Body B

Vertebrae	Compressive strength	
	Min. Value	Max. value
T-8	450	748
T-9	650	760
T-10	680	790
T-11	720	860
T-12	364	709
L-1	361	679
L-2	420	898
L-3	425	684
L-4	402	754
L-5	351	563

3. Considering only the average compressive strength, which part among the given combination is most susceptible for breaking due to an external force?

    A. T8 of body A

    B. T12 of body B

    C. T8 of body B.

    D. L3 of body B

4. Which among the following statements, can be deduced from the above data?

    A. Compressive strength of the vertebrae of both the bodies follows a definite pattern, decreasing from L-5 to T-8.

    B. Compressive strength of the vertebrae of body A only follows a definite pattern, decreasing from L-5 to T-8.

    C. Compressive strength of the vertebrae of body B only follows a definite pattern, decreasing from L-5 to T-8.

    D. Compressive strength of the vertebrae of body A follows a definite pattern, decreasing from L-5 to T-8 except at T-11.

Solution

Question 1.

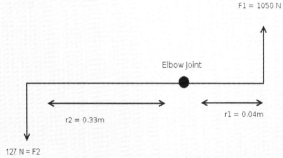

Force generated by the muscle = F1 = 1050 N
The axis of rotation of elbow joint = r1 = 0.04m
We know elbow joint is static, and the torque developed by elbow joint which is to be measured = T1
T1 = r1 × F1 = 0.04 × 1050 = 42.00 N·m , answer is A

Question 2.
If upper-limb is assessed in a mechanical device then the torque developed at elbow joint will be:

T = (r1 × F1) – (r2 × F2) = (0.04 × 1050) – (0.33 × 127) = 42.00 N·m,
Hence answer is C.

Question 3.
Step 1: Intepreting the question
Key words: Compressive strength, most susceptible and breaking.

Step 2 - Gathering Data
The table gives two values for the compressive strengths: min and max values. To solve this question, the average of these two values is taken. The values are then compared to see which has the lowest compressive strength.

Step 3 - Solution
The average of the compressive strength for T8 of body A is the average of 540 and 640 = 590. T12 of body B is 536.5, T8 of body B is 599 and L3 of body B is 554.5. Therefore the lowest compressive strength is 536.5, hence the answer is B.

Question 4.

Step 1: Intepreting the question
Key words: statements, deduce. The question only asks to deduce from the given information, not from general knowledge.

Step 2 and 3 - Gathering Data and Solution
The data from Body A and B do not follow any particular pattern, and therefore nothing can be concluded from these data sets. Hence any statements which infer a definite pattern on the WHOLE data sets must be incorrect. However D has the word "except T-11". When T-11 is taken out of the data set from Body A, then it follows a definite pattern with decreasing compressive strength from L-5 to T-11. Answer: D

Chapter 6: **Digestive tract**

> **Tip:** This topic is very rarely dealt with in the GAMSAT. The GAMSAT will ask questions on this topic indirectly. Usually the questions will involve applying the principles of osmosis and diffusion or graph reading. Have a general understanding of what the digestive system is but don't stress too much over it.

Key concepts: Digestive tract

- The gastrointestinal system is a group of organs that work to fulfil the process of absorption of nutrients
- Absorption is the transfer of *water, inorganic ions, and organic nutrients derived from the lumen of the digestive tract to the blood and the lymph*
- The process for food absorption begins in the upper digestive tract where chewing and salivary secretion prepare food for swallowing.
- The stomach is a storage organ for food which discharges its contents into the duodenum at a rate that is optimal for absorption by the small intestine
- Hydrochloric acid secreted by the stomach aids in the digestion of food and activates pepsin from the gastric mucosa and initiates the digestion of protein
- Bile secreted by the liver is stored and concentrated in the gall.
- The bile salts contained in bile play important roles in
    (1) the emulsification of fat, and
    (2) the solubilization of fat digestion products.
- The muscular movements of the small intestine facilitate digestion and absorption and move unabsorbed material into the large intestine.
- Practically all carbohydrate, protein, and lipid and most water and inorganic ions are absorbed during transit through the small intestine.
- The absorption of sodium and water is completed in the proximal large intestine. At infrequent intervals, propulsive mass movements of the proximal colon drive contents into the distal colon, where they are stored for varying periods of time
- When the rectum is distended, the defecation reflex is activated and faeces are moved to the outside of the body.

GAMSAT Style Question

Question 1.

Diarrhoea is a condition where the individual has frequent and watery bowel movements. Diarrhoea is caused when the rate of absorption is exceeded by fluid entry into the colon. Bacteria, such as cholera, are bound to the intestinal lining and release toxins that induce massive fluid secretion into the intestinal lumen. If untreated, this condition can be fatal.

Cholera toxin is composed of two sub-units: A and B sub-unit. The B sub-unit binds the toxin to the epithelial cells, while the A sub-unit inhibits the control of production of cyclic AMP, which causes a reversal in water flow. The reversal in water flow from the interstitial fluid to the lumen could be caused by

A. inhibition of Cl^- release from the crypt cell into the lumen

B. inhibition of Na^+ absorption from the lumen into the crypt cell

C. stimulation of Cl^- release from the crypt cell into the lumen

D. stimulation of Cl^- release from the crypt cell into the lumen and inhibition of Na^+ absorption into the crypt cell from the lumen

Solution

Question 1.

Step 1: Intepreting the question
The question is asking which of the four choices is the most probable cause of diarrhoea.

Step 2 and 3 - Gathering Data and Solution
During the digestive process, a large quantity of water is secreted into the lumen of the intestine. For diarrhoea to occur there must be an accumulation of water in the intestinal lumen. By osmosis we know that water follows the concentration gradient of solutes, and therefore an increase in electrolyte concentration must occur. Therefore answer A is incorrect, as it reduces the concentration of ions in the lumen. B and C are feasible as they increase lumen concentration of ions, however D is the correct answer, as both the inhibition of Na^+ absorption and increased secretion of Cl^- into the lumen would cause the greatest amount of electrolyte accumulation in the intestinal lumen, and hence the greatest amount of water would be secreted into the bowel.

Chapter 7: **Respiratory and Circulatory system**

Key concepts: Gas exchange in animals

- Gas exchange ensures cellular respiration by supplying oxygen (O_2) and removing a by-product, carbon dioxide (CO_2) from the body of animals
- Involves the movement of gases between the environment and mitochondria-the site of cellular respiration
- In unicellular organisms, O_2 reaches mitochondria simply by diffusing through the plasma membrane and cytosol while in multicellular organisms, diffusion is usually inadequate and a variety of mechanisms have evolved in these higher organisms to ensure an adequate supply of O_2 and removal of CO_2.
- Animals inhabit a diverse array of habitats and usually terrestrial animals obtain their O_2 from the atmosphere, while aquatic animals extract O_2 from water.

> *Tip:* There is likely to be questions in the GAMSAT about oxygen usage in both animals and humans. It is useful to know basic concepts such as oxygen metabolism and respiration.

GAMSAT Style Questions

Question (1-2).

Below is a model showing the ventilator system of fish. Most fish actively ventilate their gills by a double pump action involving sequential contractions and expansions of buccal and operculum cavities. Gills present a resistance to water flow between the two chambers. The mouth and the operculum effectively operate as valves. During inspiration, the mouth opens and the operculum remains closed. On expiration, the mouth closes and the operculum opens forcing water out of both cavities.

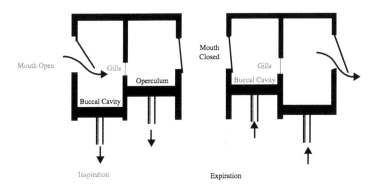

1. From the diagram, hydrostatic pressure across the gills of a fish is

   A. lower in the operculum cavity than the buccal cavity during expiration
   B. higher in the operculum cavity than the buccal cavity during inspiration
   C. is maintained across the gills throughout the entire respiration process
   D. higher in the buccal cavity than the operculum cavity during expiration

2. In some fish such as tuna and shark, ventilation is powered by locomotory muscles and does not require additional work of muscle for the fish's respiratory system. What would occur if these fishes were to accelerate for predatory or survival purposes?

   A. The fish can accelerate to faster swimming speeds without expending more energetic cost for swimming
   B. The fish would have less oxygen intake due to water moving through the gills faster at an increased speed
   C. The fish would expend more energy on respiration
   D. There would be no increase or decrease in the energy requirements of the fish

Question (3-4).

In "Closed Circuit Spirometry" the subject breathes and re-breathes from a spirometer filled with 100% oxygen. Since the subject is only allowed to breathe the air in the spirometer with no access to ambient air, this is considered a closed system.

Carbon dioxide in the exhaled air is absorbed by a canister of absorbent placed in the breathing circuit. A drum attached to the spirometer revolves at a known speed. As the volume of the spirometer decreases, a pen records this change on graph paper attached to the drum.

The subject's oxygen consumption is calculated as the difference between the starting and end points marked on the pen recording system reflecting the change in the volume of air in the spirometer drum.

The diagram below represents a spirometry tracing illustrating the changes in lung volume that occurred when a subject inhaled maximally and then rapidly exhaled as much gas as possible.

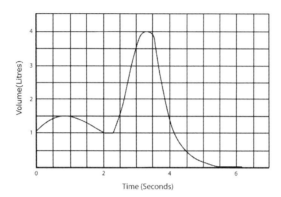

3. If the patient's total lung capacity is 6 L, what is the functional residual capacity?

    A. 1L
    B. 2L
    C. 3L
    D. 4L

4. What is the inspiratory capacity?

    A. 1.0L
    B. 2.0L
    C. 2.5L
    D. 3.0L

Question 5.

High altitude adaptation is a complex physiological process that involves an increase in both the amount of haemoglobin per erythrocyte and in the number of erythrocytes. The consequent decrease in O_2-binding affinity, as indicated by its elevated P_{50}, increases the amount of O_2 that haemoglobin unloads in the capillaries. Increases in 2,3- diphosphoglyceric acid (DPG) concentration occur in individuals suffering from disorders that limit the oxygenation of the blood (hypoxia) such as various anaemia and cardiopulmonary insufficiency.

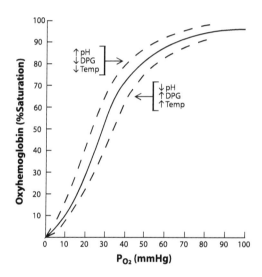

5. What would be a reasonable explanation for the increase in off-loading of O_2 at high altitudes?

    A. High altitude adaptation increases the DPG concentration in erythrocytes, which shifts the O_2 dissociation curve of Hb to right.
    B. High altitude increases the respiration rate and hence more oxygen is off-loaded to the tissues
    C. High altitude adaptation shifts the oxyhemoglobin curve to the left and increases haemoglobin concentration in erythrocytes
    D. None of the above

Question (6-8).

We need a constant supply of oxygen in order to stay alive. We use oxygen to break down food to release energy and produce carbon dioxide as a waste product. We need to continually take in oxygen from the air and expel carbon dioxide into the air.
The respiratory system functions to filter, warm, and humidify the air we breathe, and to supply cells with oxygen while removing carbon dioxide. Air moves into the lungs through the trachea and then back out again. When each breath is completed, the lung still has some air, called the residual volume. Each inhalation adds additional air. Each exhalation removes about the same volume as was inhaled.

Volume or capacity is measured in litres (l), millilitres (ml) and cubic centimetres (cm₃). One ml is equal to 1 cm^3.

The amount (volume / capacity) of air in the lungs can be measured several ways:

TOTAL LUNG CAPACITY – the amount of air in the lungs after a deep inhalation; The vital capacity plus the residual volume.

RESIDUAL LUNG CAPACITY – the amount of air left in the lungs after a deep exhalation

VITAL LUNG CAPACITY – the amount of air exhaled in one breath; The maximum amount of air that can be forcibly exhaled after breathing in as much as possible.

TIDAL LUNG CAPACITY – The amount of air your lungs hold during normal breathing; the amount of air moved in and out of the body in one breath

Two experiments are conducted as per the following procedures.

Experiment 1
1. Inject air into a plastic bag measure the volume and recode the data.
2. Inhale normally from the bag and measure the volume.
3. Record the difference in the volume
4. Repeat for a total of 5 measurements. Record the data and find the average of the measurements.

Experiment 2
Repeat all the steps of experiment 1, only this time inhale and exhale as much air as you can.

6. The final parameter measured in Experiment 1 is

    A. total lung capacity

    B. residual lung capacity

    C. vital lung capacity

    D. tidal lung capacity

7. The parameter measured in Experiment 2 is

    A. total lung capacity

    B. residual lung capacity

    C. vital lung capacity

    D. tidal lung capacity

Use the following additional information for Question 8.
A balloon was used instead of a plastic bag to measure the lung volume. The graph given below is used for converting balloon diameter into lung volume.

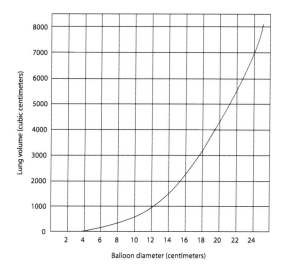

8. If a student happened to make an error of +12.5%, while measuring balloon diameters of 16 centimetres, the corresponding percentage error (approximate value) in lungs volume is,

    A. 12.5%

    B. 25%

    C. 100%

    D. 50%

Solution

Question 1.
Step 1: Intepreting the question
Key words: hydrostatic pressure and gills. Compare the hydrostatic pressure in the chambers between inspiration and expiration.

Steps 2 and 3 - Gathering Data and Solution
During inspiration, both cavities apply a negative pressure so that water can enter both the mouth and the gills. Hydrostatic pressure is needed to force water across the gills from the buccal cavity through to the operculum. During expiration and inspiration, positive and negative pressure is applied to both cavities respectively, and hence hydrostatic pressure across the gills is never reversed in direction. Hence, pressure is maintained across the gills throughout respiration.

Answer C.

Question 2.
Step 1: Intepreting the question
Key words: acceleration and respiration.

Steps 2 and 3 - Gathering Data and Solution
When the fish accelerates, the energy spent on locomotion automatically also increases the respiratory intake. Hence no extra energy has to be spent on respiration. A is incorrect, as energy is required for acceleration, regardless of respiratory process.

B is incorrect, even though water moving through the gills at a faster rate may decrease the rate of absorption; it does not reduce the total oxygen intake (as it is compensated by increased water flow).

D is incorrect, as an increase in energy requirement is needed for acceleration. Therefore by deduction, the answer is C. More energy is spent on respiration indirectly by increased locomotion, as locomotion may be seen as a form of respiration.

Question 3.

Step 1: Intepreting the question
Key words: total lung capacity and functional residual capacity.

Steps 2 and 3 - Gathering Data and Solution
Functional residual capacity is total volume of gas that is present in the lung after resting expiration. Total capacity is total volume of gas present after maximal inspiration. Therefore functional residual capacity is total lung capacity minus inspiratory capacity (see below). Therefore the answer is 6L (total) – 3L (inspiratory capacity) = 3L.

The answer is C.

Question 4.

Step 1: Intepreting the question
Key word: inspiratory capacity.

Steps 2 and 3 - Gathering Data and Solution
Inspiratory capacity is the largest volume of gas that can be inspired from resting expiratory levels. Resting expiratory levels are 1L, and maximum inspiratory level is 4L, hence inspiratory capacity is 3L.

Answer is D.

Question 5.

Step 1: Intepreting the question
Key words: off-loading O_2 and high altitude.

Steps 2 and 3 - Gathering Data and Solution
Increases in DPG would shift the O_2 dissociation curve to the right (see above figure), which would increase dissociation of O_2 from haemoglobin. Hence A would be a reasonable explanation. Higher respiration rate compensates for decreased oxygen intake, and would not necessarily result in increased O_2 concentrations in tissue, therefore B is incorrect.

Shifting the oxyhemoglobin curve to the left would result in increased binding of O_2 to haemoglobin, and result in reduced O_2 dissociation into the tissue, and would therefore represent an invalid explanation (answer C).

Therefore A is the correct answer.

Question 6.

Step 1: Intepreting the question
This is just a simple question of logic. The question is asking us to link a given parameter to one of the definitions given in the passage. The parameter here is the measurement for a "normal inhalation"

Steps 2 and 3 – Gathering the Data and Solution
The measurement here is the normal inhalation and corresponds to answer D; the tidal lung capacity.

Question 7.

Steps 1, 2 and 3
As above. The answer is the "vital lung capacity", C.

Question 8.

Step 1: Intepreting the question
This question is asking you to read straight from the graph and obtain a "percentile change"

Step 2 - Gathering Data
See graph. Adding 12.5% to 16, we get 18. This represent a change of 1000 units on the y-axis.

Step 3: Solve the problem
The corresponding change in the y-axis is 1000 units. There is a 50% error. The answer is D

Chapter 8: **Circulatory System**

- Internal to the cell, movement of ions and proteins and other intracellular particles occurs by diffusion. Diffusion can also occur from cell to cell, but it is a slow process that can only transport substances effectively over a relatively short distance. Thus, the only animals that rely exclusively on diffusion are small or thin.
- Larger animals need circulatory systems that speed the internal transport of materials.

> *Tip:* **GAMSAT questions on this topic frequently arise. Learn technical jargon such as "arterial" and "venous flow". Knowing the jargon in this topic will help you isolate the key points in any GAMSAT passage and allow you to understand the requirements for the question much faster.**

Key concepts: Circulation

- Brings dissolved substances close enough to cells or exchange surfaces so that diffusion can be effective
- It enhances diffusion
- Circulatory systems have three general functions.
  - They provide the large movement of bodily material and blood cells required throughout the body
  - The movement of heat between different parts of the body eg. to the external surface of the body from the internal surfaces.
  - A cardiovascular system that provides sufficient convective transport of O_2. Therefore, levels of respiratory gases in the blood are important factors in regulation of cardiovascular function.

Key concepts: Oxygen transport and the role of blood

In order to use oxygen, aerobic organisms must overcome:
1. The low aqueous solubility of oxygen (about 1 mM)
2. Its slow diffusion rate (oxygen will travel about 0.06 mm in one second by diffusion).
   - Large, aerobic organisms solve these problems by using haemoglobin in the blood to increase oxygen solubility and by pumping the blood to all parts of the body using the circulatory system (heart, lungs, and blood vessels).

- Heme is responsible for the characteristic red colour of blood and is the site at which each globin monomer binds one molecule of O2.
- Haemoglobin transports oxygen from the lungs, gills, or skin of an animal to its capillaries for use in respiration.

Key concepts: The human heart

- The right and left hearts (anatomically, the right and left ventricles) are connected in series, but are folded together to form a single unit
- The right heart pumps blood only to the lungs; its output is low pressure (25 mm Hg)
- The left heart pumps blood to the rest of the body; its output is high pressure (120 mm Hg)
- Because the 2 hearts are attached they beat in synchrony
- The 2 atria receive the incoming blood and pump extra blood into the ventricles
- The 2 ventricles produce enough pressure to push blood through the pulmonary and systemic circulations

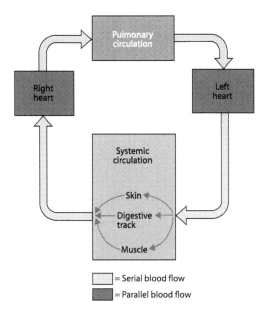

GAMSAT Style Questions

Question (1-3).

The diagram below demonstrates the blood supply to the body. The systemic circulation begins with the aorta that receives all the blood the heart pumps out. As it branches, it divides into smaller arteries, arterioles and capillaries and then returns to the heart via the venules, veins and the vena cava. The pulmonary circulation collects oxygen from the lungs to distribute to the whole body via the blood and a molecule to which the oxygen attaches called haemoglobin.

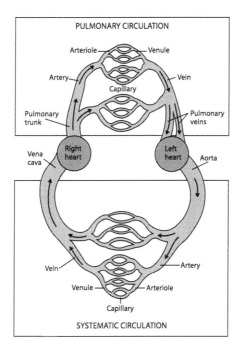

1. How many major blood vessels immediately carry blood away from the heart?

   A. 1
   B. 2
   C. 3
   D. 4

2. What would be the order of points that have the largest amount of oxygen to the least amount of the oxygen?

    A. Pulmonary trunk, Pulmonary veins, Aorta

    B. Aorta, Arteriole, Arteries

    C. Veins, Vena Cava, Pulmonary Artery, Pulmonary Vein

    D. Pulmonary Vein, Arteriole, Venule

3. The amount of haemoglobin in the Aorta compared to the Pulmonary Trunk is the

    A. same,

    B. more,

    C. less

    D. cannot be determined

Solution

Question 1.

Step 1: Intepreting the question
Key words: immediately, away and how many. The word immediately suggests urgency or "as soon as possible".

Steps 2 and 3 - Gathering Data and Solution
Ask yourself "what is the diagram telling me". It seems that the circulation of the human body has two pathways, the "pulmonary" (lungs) and "systemic" (other body systems). This assumes that you know that the heart consists of the left and right heart which act together to supply the whole body. The diagram shows the right heart pumping blood to the lungs and the left heart pumping blood to the peripheries. From the right heart stems the "pulmonary trunk" and the left stems the "aorta". Answer B.

Question 2.

Step 1: Intepreting the question
This is another order question. Note that it is asking for the "largest" to the "least". Looking at the possible answers you could ask yourself in different words, "which vessels contain how much oxygen?"

Steps 2 and 3 - Gathering Data and Solution
We are told that "pulmonary circulation collect oxygen from the lungs" for distribution. Blood that has just collected oxygen has come from the lungs through to the pulmonary veins, left heart, aorta then to the systemic circulation in the direction of the arrows in the diagram. It is logical that more oxygen will be contained in vessels that arise from the lungs. Answer is D. Use the process of elimination it cannot be the pulmonary trunk so that eliminates A, it is definitely not the veins so it leaves us with either B or D. More closely it is D.

Question 3.

Step 1: Intepreting the question
A value on the amount of "haemoglobin" compared to different vessels in the diagram.

Steps 2 and 3 - Gathering Data and Solution
If you didn't already know, haemoglobin is an oxygen-carrying molecule in the blood that is essential for life in mammals. It is already said in the passage that haemoglobin does this function. We would infer that if haemoglobin was the carrying molecule in the blood then there would be an even distribution around the body. It would "pick up" oxygen at the lungs and "drop it off" at various locations around the body. Just like a train or taxi picks up people and drops them off. The number of trains and taxis remains the same in the city but the number of people it carries differs depending on other factors. Therefore A.

Chapter 9: **Blood Pressure**

—> *Quick Facts: Blood Pressure*

- Is the force that blood exerts against the blood vessel walls.
- Results when that flow is met by resistance from vessel walls.
- Is expressed in millimetres of mercury (mm Hg). For example a blood pressure of 120mm Hg is equivalent to a pressure exerted by a column of mercury 120 mm high.

Key concepts: Diastolic and Systolic Blood Pressure

Blood Pressure Graph

- Systolic pressure is the maximum pressure exerted by the blood against the artery walls. It is the result of ventricular systole or contraction. It is normally about 120 mm Hg.

Diastolic Pressure

- Diastolic pressure is the lowest pressure in the artery. It's a result of ventricular diastole (relaxation) and is usually around 80 mm Hg.

Pulse Pressure

- Pulse Pressure is the difference between systolic and diastolic pressure.
- It's the throb you feel when you take your pulse.
  Pulse Pressure = Systolic Pressure - Diastolic Pressure
  i.e. 40 mm Hg = 120 mm Hg - 80 mm Hg

Mean Arterial Pressure (MAP)

- Mean Arterial Pressure (MAP) is a calculated "average" pressure in the arteries.
- Mean Arterial Pressure (MAP) = Diastolic Pressure + 1/3 Pulse Pressure
- MAP is closer to the diastolic pressure than systolic pressure because the heart stays longer in diastole
- MAP is the force that propels the blood through the arteries.

Blood Pressure Sounds

- When blood pressure is measured, a cuff is inflated to constrict an artery so that no blood flows through. Since the pressure in the cuff is greater than the pressure in the artery, the artery is closed off and no blood flows through.

- As the cuff pressure is gradually released, but the artery is still partially constricted, blood flow resumes. Sounds can be heard with a stethoscope because the blood flows turbulently, causing audible sounds.
- When enough pressure is released to fully open the artery, the blood flows freely and the sounds disappear because smooth flowing blood does not create sounds

Checking Blood Pressure

- The first sounds that are heard indicate systolic pressure. When the sounds stop, diastolic pressure has been reached.

--> *Quick Facts: Blood Pressure*

- Systolic pressure = highest pressure in an artery; result of ventricular contraction
- Diastolic pressure = lowest pressure in an artery; result of ventricular relaxation
- Pulse pressure = systolic pressure - Diastolic Pressure
- Mean Arterial Pressure (MAP) = Diastolic pressure + 1/3 Pulse pressure
- When blood pressure is measured, first sounds indicate systolic pressure; end of sounds indicates diastolic pressure

GAMSAT Style Questions

Question 1.

The graph below demonstrates a normal cardiac output curve. The curve starts at a slightly negative right atrial pressure (remember that negative pressure just means sub atmospheric) and projects upward and to the right. Its exact position for use in qualitative analysis is not critical. The normal cardiac output is 5 L/min. The axes of these curves are such that the y-axis is cardiac output and the x- axis is right atrial pressure.

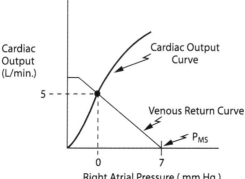

1. Administration of an inotropic agent will increase contractility of the heart making it "hyper effective". What effect would this have on the cardiac output curve in the graph?

   A. Will shift the cardiac output curve up and to the left.
   B. Shift the curve up and to the right
   C. Shift the curve down and left
   D. Shift the curve down and right.

Question 2.

The vertebrate circulatory system is essentially a pump that pushes blood through a system of biological tubing. It works against a resistance that is caused by the vessels of the body. In an analogy, it is very similar to "Ohms Law" which states that the Voltage power supply) is proportional to the resistance of the circuit $(V = IR)$. In the case of blood flow, the difference in pressure $\Delta P(P_a-P_v)$ is proportional to the resistance of the peripheries. So $\Delta P = V_b R$ where V_b is the rate of blood flow.

In Figure 1 below, this represents an analogy of the heart and circulatory system to a pump.

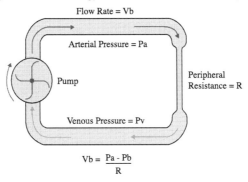

Figure 1

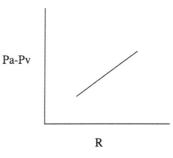

Figure 2

2. Figure 2 shows the graph of a "normal" healthy person. In a person with high blood pressure, what could be the possible graphical representation?

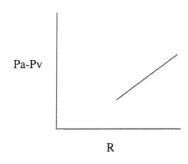

A.

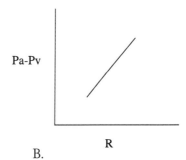

B.

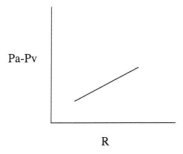

C.

D. Both A and B

Question 3.

This is a simplistic model of a circulatory system. In a closed circulatory system, a heart distributes blood carrying essential nutrients to the body's peripheries first via an arterial system and returning via a venous system.

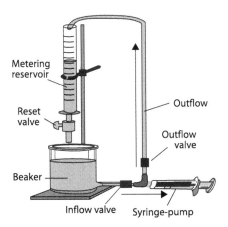

Figure 1

3. In Figure 1 which item could represent the heart, venous system and arterial system respectively.

    A. Syringe-Pump, inflow valve, outflow valve

    B. Syringe-Pump, Beaker, Metering Reservoir

    C. Syringe Pump, metering reservoir, inflow valve

    D. Syringe Pump, outflow valve, inflow valve

Solution

Question 1.

<u>Step 1: Intepreting the question</u>
Key words: increase contractility and cardiac output. The question asks what effect increased heart rate has on cardiac output and its relationship to right ventricular pressure.

<u>Steps 2 and 3 - Gathering Data and Solution</u>
We know that increased contractility means increased cardiac output and therefore the curve shifts up in the graph. Hence answers C and D are incorrect. Increased contractility of the heart results in a reduced end-systolic volume in the ventricle as the heart is contracting more strongly and for a longer duration. Because the ventricle is emptying faster, the atrium can fill the ventricle more under similar pressures, which would shift the curve to the left.

Hence the correct answer is A

Question 2.

Try doing this one yourself, writing out your own three-step method.

Answer: D

Question 3.

<u>Step 1: Intepreting the question</u>
Key words: heart, venous system and arterial system.

<u>Steps 2 and 3 - Gathering Data and Solution</u>
The easiest way to solve this question is to go through the choices. The heart is the syringe pump, and it is listed in all four choices. The venous system is defined as anything that flows to the heart, while the arterial systems is anything system that flows away from the heart. Therefore everything from the outflow valve to the reset valve is the arterial system, while from the beaker to the inflow valve is the venous system.

Hence the correct answer is A

Chapter 10: **Immune system**

Key concepts: Immune system

- Organisms must be able to defend themselves against micro-organisms and parasites. It is at this level that the immune system is of key importance in defence.
- The role of the immune system is to provide protection against viruses, bacteria, fungi and other small parasites, and any other macromolecular organic matter that threatens the integrity of the organism
- The mammalian immune system is studied, primarily because it is among the most complex and advanced but also because it is the best understood
- There are four important concepts
    - Substances that an immune system reacts against, for example, molecules on the surface of a bacterium are called antigens.
    - The cells in the body that carry out many of the functions of the immune system are lymphocytes. There are two main types: B lymphocytes and T lymphocytes.
    - B lymphocytes make and release antibodies, which are important defence molecules that react with and destroy antigens.
    - T lymphocytes regulate immune responses and can directly attack and kill foreign organisms or infected cells.

GAMSAT Style Question

Question 1.

The human body's defence mechanism against micro-organisms consists of the "Immune System" and the "Immune Response". A foreign body labelled with an "antigen" enters the body, results in the formation of a corresponding antibody against the invading organism. A key part of specific immunity involves immunological memory. For instance when an individual comes into contact with polio virus, the immune system remembers this and if the person comes into contact with the polio virus again a secondary response occurs. The graph below represents an antibody response to "Salmonella Typh" in an inoculated mouse.

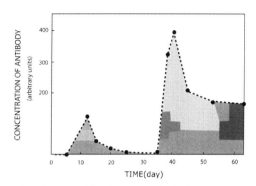

1. According to the graph when would it be most likely that the antigen was introduced into the mouse?

    A. Day 1 and 43

    B. Day 25 and 50

    C. Day 1 and 34

    D. Day 13 and 43

Solution

Question 1.

Step 1: Intepreting the question
Key words: graph, antigen and likely. The question asks us to make an assumption based on the data.

Steps 2 and 3 - Gathering Data and Solution
The graph shows two responses to the introduction of an antigen. One on the 5th day and the other on the 34th day. The second response to the same antigen will always be greater than the first one. Furthermore, the first response is always delayed by a couple of days before the response becomes evident. Therefore the mouse was probably injected with the antigen a couple of days before response one (which would be equivalent to day 1). A second response to the same antigen is immediate because the immune system "remembers". Therefore the second time the antigen was introduced would be at 34 days. The answer is C.

Chapter 11: Endocrine system

Functions of the Endocrine System

The main functions of the endocrine system include regulation of:
- Water balance.
- Uterine contractions during parturition.
- Milk release from the breasts.
- Metabolism.
- Tissue maturation.
- Sodium, potassium, and calcium ion concentration of blood.
- Heart rate.
- Blood pressure.
- Preparation for physical activity.
- Blood glucose concentration.
- Immune cell production.
- Reproductive functions in males and females.

→Quick Facts: Chemical Signals

- Chemical signals bind to receptor sites on receptor molecules.
- Intracellular chemical signals are produced in one part of a cell and travel to another part of the same cell and bind to receptors.
- Intercellular chemical signals are released from one cell, are carried in the intercellular fluid, and bind to receptors in other cells.
- Intercellular chemical signals can be classified as autocrine, paracrine, hormone, neurohormone, neuromodulator, neurotransmitter, or pheromone chemical signals.

Receptors
- Chemical signals bind to receptor sites on receptor molecules to produce a response.
- Intracellular receptors are located in the cytoplasm or nuclei and can regulate enzyme activity or regulate the synthesis of specific messenger RNA.
- Membrane-bound receptors can produce a response by directly opening ion channels, activating G proteins, or activating enzymes that synthesize intracellular chemical signals or by phosphorylating proteins inside of the cell.

Hormones

- Endocrine glands produce hormones that are released into the circulatory system and travel some distance, where they act on target tissues to produce a response.
- A target tissue for a given hormone has receptor molecules for that hormone.
- Hormones are basically proteins, peptides, or lipids.
- Protein and peptide hormones bind to receptors on the cell membrane and cause permeability changes or the production of a second messenger inside the cell. Lipid-soluble hormones, such as the steroids and thyroid hormones, enter the cell and bind to receptors inside the cell.
- The combining of hormones with their receptors results in a response.

Regulation of Hormone Secretion

- The secretion of hormones is controlled by negative-feedback mechanisms.
- Secretion of hormones from a specific gland is controlled by blood levels of some chemicals, another hormone or nervous system.
- The endocrine system consists of ductless glands.
- Some glands of the endocrine system perform more than one function.

AMSAT Style Question

Question 1.

In the human body, homeostasis or regulation of bodily functions is maintained by the endocrine system. The adrenal glands are located above the kidneys and release cortical hormones which have many functions such as regulating the inflammatory system and coping with stress level. The diagram shows what is called a "negative feedback mechanism" which aids in controlling levels of cortical hormone in the body. When too much cortical hormone is produced, the hypothalamus reacts by releasing substances that decrease the amount of cortical substances.

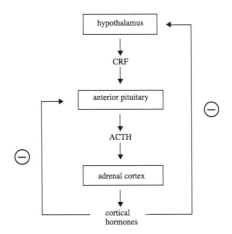

1. A person who has an autoimmune inflammatory disorder such as rheumatoid arthritis may be on long-term corticosteroids to decrease their symptoms. Corticosteroids act in a similar fashion to the cortical hormones produced by the adrenal glands. According to the diagram what would occur in the long term?

    A. CRF will increase while ACTH will increase

    B. ACTH will increase while CRF will decrease

    C. CRF and ACTH will both increase

    D. CRF and ACTH will both decrease

Solution

Question 1.

Step 1: Intepreting the question
Key words: corticosteroids and long term

Steps 2 and 3 - Gathering Data and Solution
We know that corticosteroids are cortical hormones. Furthermore, we know that cortical hormones have an inhibitory effect on the hypothalamus and anterior pituitary to release CRF and ACTH (see diagram above). Therefore long-term application of corticosteroids would result in long-term suppression of these two hormones. Hence the answer is D.

Chapter 12: **Nervous system**

Key concepts: Nervous system

- The nervous system is divided into the central nervous system (CNS) and the peripheral nervous system (PNS).
  - The central nervous system includes the brain and spinal cord, which contain nuclei and tracts.
  - The peripheral nervous system consists of nerves and ganglia.

Key concepts: Neurons

- A neuron consists of dendrites, a cell body and an axon.
- The cell body contains the nucleus, Nissl bodies, neurofibrils and other organelles.
- Dendrites receive stimuli, and the axon conducts nerve impulses away from the cell body.
- A nerve is a collection of axons in the PNS.
- A sensory, or afferent, neuron is pseudounipolar and conducts impulses from sensory receptors into the CNS.
- A motor, or efferent, neuron is multipolar and conducts impulses from the CNS to effector organs.
- Interneurons, or association neurons, are located entirely within the CNS.
- Somatic motor nerves innervate skeletal muscle; autonomic nerves innervate smooth muscle, cardiac muscle, and glands.

AMSAT Style Questions

Question (1-4).

The human sensory and motor system consists of nerve cells travelling centrally to and from the peripheries to certain areas of the brain. Within the last century, to represent the distribution of sensation and motor control in the brain, neuroscientists have developed the "homunculus" which displays the location of the cortical representation of the various parts of the human body through a cross section of the brain. In the diagram below, two homunculus have been shown, one for sensory distribution and one for motor distribution. The size of the various parts is proportionate to the area devoted to them.

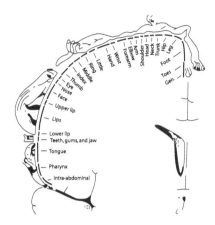
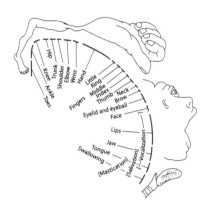

Sensory Homunculus   *Motor Homunculus*

1. From the diagram, where would pain, thermal and tactile sensations from the peripheries be felt the most?

    A. Head
    B. Hands and Fingers
    C. Feet and Legs
    D. Arms and Elbows

2. In what order would be the most sensitive areas of the body to the least?

    A. Lips, Face, Fingers, Hand
    B. Genitals, Hip, Face, Nose
    C. Lips, Face, Genitals, Neck
    D. Neck, Hand, Face, Lips

3. Out of the following, which has the most motor coordination according to the diagram?

    A. Knee
    B. Lips
    C. Hand
    D. Tongue

4. Which of the following lists below ranks the body parts from the least motor coordination to the most?

    A. Hip, Face, Knee, Hand

    B. Hip, Knee, Ankle, Hand

    C. Lips, Knee, Hip, Neck

    D. Face, Hand, Fingers, Toes

Question (5-6).

This diagram shows different senses and the distribution to various aspects of the human brain. The brain stem is an intermediate area where nervous signals are relayed to and from the brains higher centres.

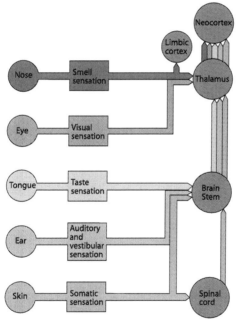

5. Which of the following systems has the most direct pathway to the higher centres in the brain?

    A. Tongue and Ear

    B. Nose and Eye

    C. Nose and Tongue

    D. Skin

6. If an individual had damage to the brain stem from a motor vehicle accident, which sensations out of the following would have the highest probability of being affected?

    A. Smell

    B. Touch

    C. Taste

    D. Cannot be determined from the given information

Solution

Question 1

Step 1: Intepreting the question

Underline the key words. In this case they would be "pain", "thermal" and "tactile". The question asks specifically "where" and from the answers we can gauge that this refers to certain parts of the human body. Therefore to rephrase the question simply we would say something like: Which parts of the body has the largest supply of nerves for sensation?

NB: Do not let words which you may not be sure of distract you. Whatever it is in the GAMSAT, you can always simplify what is being asked in any science question so you can answer conclusively.

Steps 2 and 3 - Gathering Data and Solution

From the passage it specifically says that this has something to do with nerve distribution. The key to answering this question lies in the last sentence "the size of the various parts is proportionate to the area devoted to them". Looking at the diagram, we can see that that the body parts shown are grossly disproportionate to what they are in the human body. From the passage it means that the areas of which they are represented to them in the brain are "proportionate" to the area devoted to them. Knowing this point we can answer the questions.

First of all, we are talking about sensations so out of both diagrams we would obviously choose the first "sensory homunculus". We are asked to find the largest area of representation in the body. Looking at the diagram the entire head seems to be the part of the body represented the most.

Hence the answer is A.

Question 2

Step 1: Intepreting the question
Key words: Order, most, least and sensitive. In these questions where we are asked to place a list in order, it is imperative that we understand which order as a lot of good students will get the order correct but in the opposite direction.

Steps 2 and 3 - Gathering Data and Solution
Use the process of elimination in this question. We know that the question asks from the "most" to "least" so we can already gauged that A or C **wo**uld be a good option. In A we can see that the Hand is placed last and on the diagram the hand has a relatively large area of distribution.

The answer is therefore C.

Question 3

Step 1: Intepreting the question
Key words: most and motor co-ordination. The question's key point is "which body part has the largest distribution of nerves to the head?".

Steps 2 and 3 - Gathering Data and Solution
Look for the largest line in the "motor homunculus".

Thus it is the Hand, C.

Question 4

Step 1: Intepreting the question
Place a list of items in order from "least" to the "most".

Steps 2 and 3 - Gathering Data and Solution
Use elimination again to narrow down to two possible answers. In this case it would seem to be either A or B because the "hip" seems to be least represented in the cortex.

Therefore after more analysis we would say B.

Question 5

<u>Step 1: Intepreting the question</u>
Key words: direct, brain and higher centre.

<u>Steps 2 and 3 - Gathering Data and Solution</u>
Schematic displays various senses to the higher centres in the brain via the brain stem and spinal cord. The nose and eye are seen to directly enter the thalamus in the brain. Some have suggested that that the optic and olfactory nerves are not part of the cranial nervous system because they are direct projections from the brain itself and are highly specialised structures that are embryologically different to other cranial nerves.

Answer B.

Question 6

<u>Step 1: Intepreting the question</u>
Key words: brain stem, sensation and accident. With accident the question implies loss of function of that particular area/pathway.

<u>Steps 2 and 3 - Gathering Data and Solution</u>
Damage to the brain stem would result in all function downstream from the brain stem to be non-functional. Smell is upstream from the brain stem, so it is least likely to be affected.

For the somatic sensation, the brain stem receives stimuli both directly and through the spinal cord which are then integrated within the brain stem. Therefore, at least 2 parts of the brain stem are involved in processing this information. Any damage to the brain stem is likely to damage the delicate balance of coordinating the inputs.

Taste sensation is processed directly in the brain stem, so probably a smaller part of the brain stem is involved, therefore it will probably be less likely to be affected if the extent of the damage to the brainstem is unknown.

Therefore the answer is B.

Chapter 13: **Molecular Genetics**

Key concepts: DNA

- Information in a cell is stored in the nucleus in the form of DNA. DNA is used by the cell as a blueprint to create proteins and thereby create structural and functional entities that make cells viable.

- Under resting circumstances, DNA is double stranded, consisting of a pair of strands which consist of nucleotides. These strands are held together by hydrogen bonds, which can be broken either enzymatically, or through heat.

- Information is stored by DNA in a sequence of the nucleotides. Nucleotides are nitrogenous bases. There are four nucleotides present in DNA: adenosine (A), thymine (T), cytosine (C) and guanine (G).

- Each amino acid present in the cell is encoded by a *triplet* of nucleotides. Therefore a strand of *triplet* nucleotides would represent a strand of amino acid after *transcription* and *translation*. The end product is a peptide, which is a building block of the cell.

- *Transcription* is a process where parts of the DNA are copied to mRNA. *Translation* is the process where mRNA is used as a template to create the peptide.

- RNA is very similar to DNA, and is used for transcription. RNA has four nucleotides as DNA, with the exception of a thymine (T), it has uracil (U).

- *Transcription* is a process where the double stranded DNA molecule unwinds and is split into single stranded DNA molecules. RNA polymerase binds to a "start" codon on the single stranded DNA and copies the DNA to form mRNA until a "stop" codon is reached. The mRNA dissociates from the RNA polymerase, and the polymerase from the DNA molecule, after which the two strands of DNA reassociate to form a double stranded DNA molecule.

- mRNA binds to a ribosomal sub-unit where tRNA which has *triplet codons* complementary to the mRNA binds to the mRNA. Each tRNA is conjugated to a specific amino acid that is designated by the triplet. After the tRNA has bound to the mRNA, it dissociates but binds the amino acid to the growing peptide.

GAMSAT Style Questions

Question (1-3)

When a solution of duplex DNA is heated above a characteristic temperature, its native structure collapses and its two complementary strands separate and assume the random coil conformation.

This denaturation process is accompanied by a qualitative change in the DNA's physical properties. The most convenient way of monitoring the native state of DNA is by its ultraviolet (UV) absorbance spectrum. This phenomenon, which is known as the hyperchromic effect (Greek; *hyper,* above; *chroma,* colour), results from the disruption of the electronic interactions among nearby bases. DNA's hyperchromic shift, as monitored at a particular wavelength (usually 260 nm), occurs over a narrow temperature range. This indicates that the denaturation of DNA is a cooperative phenomenon in which the collapse of one part of the structure destabilizes the remainder.

T m' is denoted as the melting temperature.

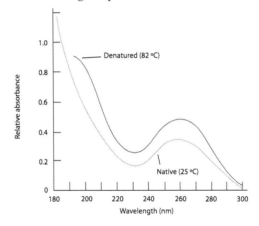

1. Which of the following statements can be inferred from the above diagram?

    A. Relative absorbance of denatured DNA is approximately 100% greater than the native DNA at 230 nm
    B. Relative absorbance of denatured DNA is approximately 100% greater than the native DNA at 210 nm
    C. Relative absorbance of denatured DNA is approximately 100% greater than the native DNA at 280 nm
    D. None of these statements can be inferred

2. Among the following given temperatures, the temperature at which it is most likely that denaturing of DNA will not take place is

A. 85°C
B. 90°C
C. 83°C
D. 25°C

3. The relative absorbance of DNA at 260nm is plotted against temperature in Figure 1.

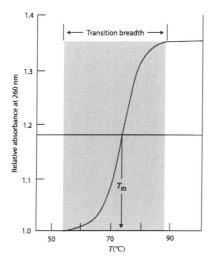

Figure 1

Which of the following facts can be inferred from Figure 1?

A. The melting temperature Tm is the temperature at which approximately 80% of maximum absorbance increase is attained.

B. The melting temperature Tm is the temperature at which approximately 50% of maximum absorbance increase is attained.

C. The melting temperature Tm is the temperature at which approximately 20% of maximum absorbance increase is attained

D. Relative absorbance is independent of temperature

Question 4.

Phylogenetic trees are used to describe the evolutionary relationships between organisms. Below is phylogenetic tree that is used to describe the relationship between the platypus, koala and dingo. The lower down the scale the more general the feature, the higher up the scale the more specific the feature.

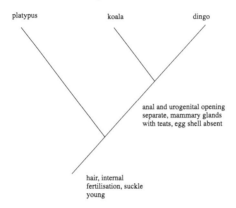

The following is an example to show how the sequence of bases in a piece of DNA can be used to discover the relationships of organism to one another. The table beneath shows the bases present in three nucleotide positions in a DNA subunit of the listed organisms. The drosophila insect has the base positions T G A in the sequences below and is furthest down the phylogenetic tree. The more differences in the DNA bases in the relative positions the further away the organism is to drosophila.

Base position	1151	2239	3988
Mouse, Mus	T	A	G
Cockatoo, Cacatua	C	G	G
Frog, Xenopus	T	G	A
Insect, Drosophila	T	G	A

3. There are 3 possible phylogenetic trees for these three vertebrates. Which one relates to the frog, mouse and cockatoo?

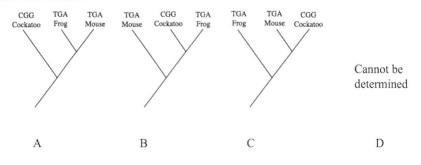

A   B   C   D

Solution

Question 1.

Step 1: Intepreting the question
To compare the absorbance of native and denatured DNA

Steps 2 and 3 - Gathering Data and Solution
The absorbance of native DNA at 230nm can be read off the graph, and is approximately 0.16. The absorbance of denatured DNA is 0.26. Therefore the absorbance is approximately 63% greater. Therefore A is incorrect. The absorbance at 210nm for native DNA is 0.38 and denatured DNA 0.65, which is about a 71% increase. Therefore B is incorrect. The absorbance at 280nm for native DNA is 0.19 and denatured DNA 0.27, which is about a 42% increase. Therefore C is incorrect.

By elimination, D is the correct answer.

Question 2.

Step 1: Intepreting the question
Key words: denaturing, temperature. The question asks at what temperature DNA denatures.

Steps 2 and 3 - Gathering Data and Solution
It follows that DNA does not denature in the body, as otherwise live would be impossible. Therefore the denaturing process has to take place above 37°C. The only temperature which is below 37°C is D.

Therefore D is the correct answer.

Question 3.

Step 1: Intepreting the question
Key words: absorbance, melting temperature.

Steps 2 and 3 - Gathering Data and Solution
The melting temperature Tm is indicated on the graph to occur at 72°C. When looking at the relative absorbance, it can be seen that this corresponds to about half of the maximum height of the graph.

Therefore B is the correct answer.

Question 4.

Step 1: Intepreting the question

The question asks for the evolutionary relationship between the three organisms listed in the table.

Step 2 - Gathering Data

-Numbers refer to position of DNA in the chain.

-1st diagram of the phylogenic tree shows that link between related organisms by the different and common characteristics that each possesses

-The insect is the furthest down the tree

Step 3: Solve the problem

Insect in TGA and frog is TGA= no differences in the DNA in the three individual positions. Cockatoo and Insect = 2 differences in the DNA positions. Therefore the frog has to be closest to the bottom and C is correct because there are no other choices where the frog is in this position.

Chapter 14: **Mendelian genetics**

> *Tip:* Question based on this topic frequently occurs in the GAMSAT. It is one of the topics you need to know well.

Key concepts: Mendel's first law: Law of segregation

Mendel postulated four principles of inheritance:
- Genes exist in alternative forms now referred to as alleles
- An organism has two alleles for each inherited trait, one inherited from each parent
- The two alleles segregate during meiosis, resulting in gametes that carry only one allele for any given inherited trait
- If two alleles of an individual organism are different, only one will be fully expressed and the other will be silent. The expressed allele is said to be dominant and the silent allele is said to be recessive. In genetics problems, dominant alleles are assigned capital letters and recessive alleles are assigned lower case letters. Organisms that contain two copies of the same allele are homozygous for that trait, organisms that carry two different alleles are heterozygous

Key concept: Punnet Square

	B	b
B	BB	bB
b	Bb	bb

This cross yields three possible genotypes in the offspring - BB, Bb, and bb.
- Punnet square also indicates how likely a particular child of this mating is to have a given genotype. In this case, there is a one in four (25%) chance that the child would be BB, two in four (50%) that it would be Bb and one in four (25%) that it would be bb.
- Thus on average, about 25% of the children of this cross should have a genotype of bb.

Punnet Squares of all possible crosses:

BB x BB	BB x Bb	Bb x Bb	Bb x bb	bb x bb
B B	B B	B b	B b	b b
B BB BB	B BB BB	B BB bB	b Bb bb	b bb **bb**
B BB BB	b Bb Bb	b Bb bb	b Bb Bb	**b** bb bb

An individual can have a genotype of BB (Homozygous dominant), Bb (Heterozygous), or b▮ (Homozygous Recessive). Any of these individuals could mate with any other, thus there ar▮ several possible crosses as shown in the Punnet Squares.

GAMSAT Style Question

Question (1-2).

In guinea-pigs, multiple genes control the colour of the fur and whether there are spots on the fur or not. Consider the colour of the fur to be controlled by one allele, and whether the fur is spotted or not by another. Plain is considered dominant, while a spotted coat is considered recessive. The colour of the coat is black when homozygous for black, yellow when heterozygous for black and white, and white when homozygous for white. Homozygous white fur is lethal, and do not survive birth.

1. When mating two yellow guinea-pigs, what is the likely proportion of off-spring?

A. All yellow
B. 3 yellow to 1 black
C. 2 yellow to 1 black
D. 1 yellow to 1 black

2. Two yellow spotted guinea pigs are mated. The phenotype would most likely be

    A. 25% black spotted

    B. 25% yellow spotted

    C. 33.33% black spotted

    D. 50% yellow plain

Solution

Question 1

Step 1: Intepreting the question
Key words: proportion and off-spring

Steps 2 and 3 - Gathering Data and Solution
When two yellow guinea pigs mate, by the punnet square, the proportions would be 25% white, 50% yellow and 25% black. Because the whites are lethal, that group can be eliminated, so the proportions now are 66% yellow and 33% black. This would be equivalent to 2 yellow for every black.

Therefore the correct answer is C.

Question 2

Step 1: Intepreting the question
The question is the same as the previous one, except now they have included one extra variable; namely whether the coat is spotted or not.

Steps 2 and 3 - Gathering Data and Solution
We know that spotted coats are recessive therefore the genotype of the guinea pigs must be homozygous for spotting. Hence, no plain coats are possible and answer D can be eliminated. By the punnet square, the proportions would be 25% white, 50% yellow and 25% black. Because the whites are lethal that group can be eliminated, so the proportions now are 66% yellow and 33% black.

Therefore answers A and B are incorrect and C is the correct answer.

Printed in Great Britain
by Amazon